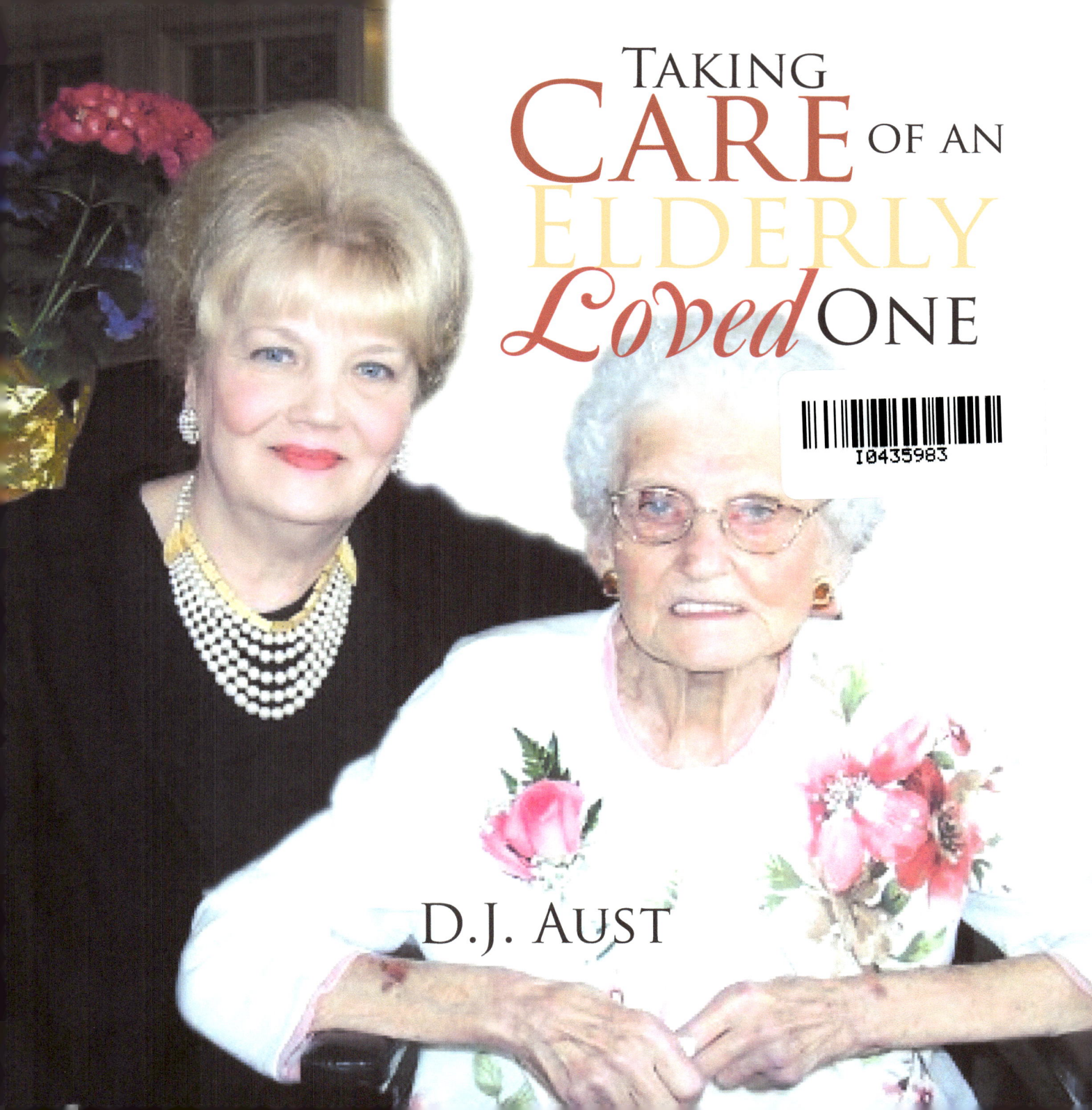

Taking CARE OF AN ELDERLY Loved ONE

D.J. Aust

Copyright © 2016 by D.J. Aust. 731685

ISBN: Softcover   978-1-5245-0267-6
         EBook   978-1-5245-0266-9

Print information available on the last page

Rev. date: 08/01/2016

To order additional copies of this book, contact:
Xlibris
1-888-795-4274
www.Xlibris.com
Orders@Xlibris.com

This book is dedicated to

my mother-in-law, Eleanor Snyder Aust,

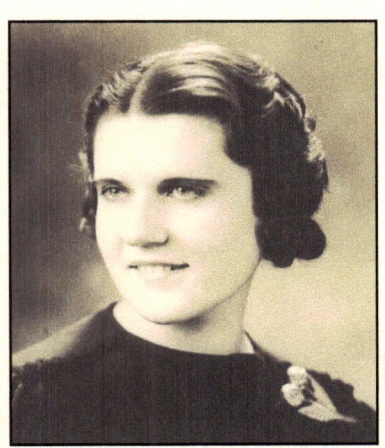

and

my mother, Helen Waligora Grabowski.

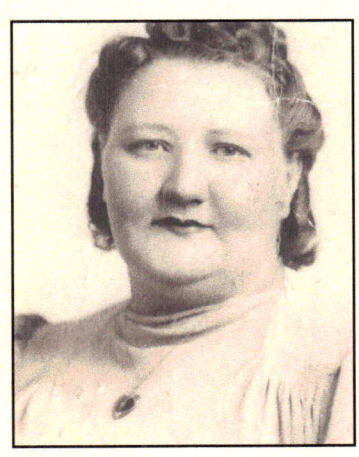

At first, when my mother-in-law came to live with us, we had no idea what was in store for us. She didn't come with instructions, and each day was a learning experience.

I hope this book will be a guide for you along your journey.

My mother-in-law was an amazing person. She was always there when we needed her. She would never say no to anyone who needed her help. She was a daughter, a sister, a wife, a mother, a cousin, a sister-in-law, a grandmother, a friend, a registered nurse, and my mother-in-law. She was good at all these roles.

She was my mother-in-law for over forty years and was so good to me. How she could have put up with me at times, I'll never know. She always said family was so important.

She was a very caring and loving person. We shared a lot of special time together, secrets, and special memories, for which I will always be grateful. She made me promise not to put her in a nursing home if she would be unable to take care of herself.

She knew I would keep my promise.

I lost my mother when I was eleven. I believe that was one of the reasons my mother-in-law was so special to me. I used to tell my husband that if I had known his mother before I married him, I would have married him because his mother was so great.

At eighty-eight, my mother-in-law, whom I will now refer to as Mom, had a stroke that affected part of her memory. Not long after that, my father-in-law died, and Mom lived alone in their home.

Mom was a very independent person and wanted to stay in her own home. We tried respecting her wishes, but when her doctor told us she could no longer live alone, we knew something had to be done. He also said, if she wasn't living with someone by her next appointment, he would have a social worker admit her into a nursing home. It was then that I knew it was time to keep my promise.

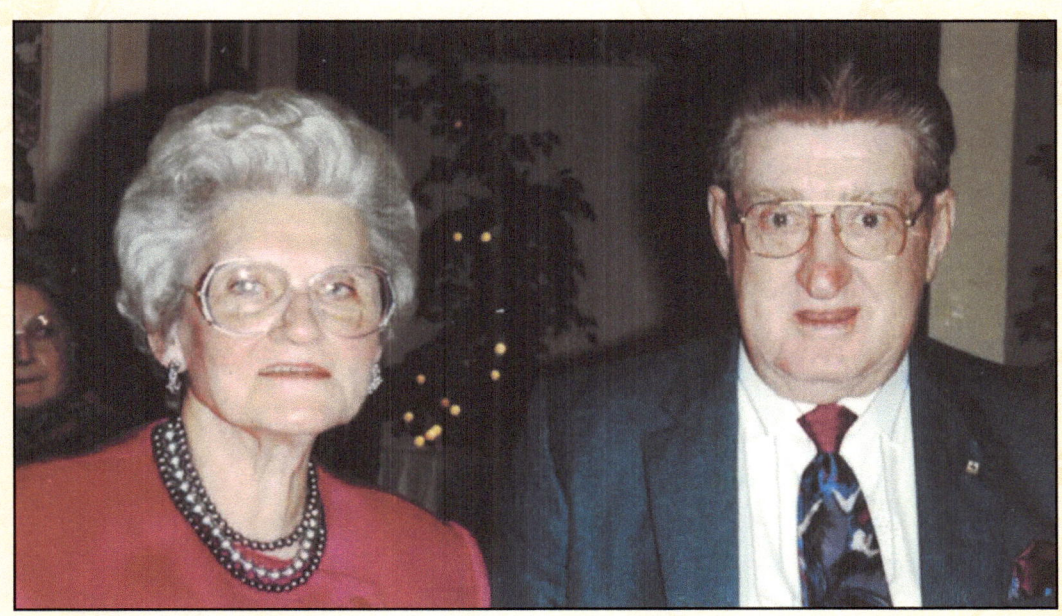

Mom and Dad

The following weekend, my husband and I brought her out to our home and asked her to stay for a few days. This was very hard for all of us because Mom didn't want to rely on us and wanted to live independently. Eventually, over time, it all worked out.

I would ask Mom from time to time if she wanted to go into a nursing home with people her own age. She would always say "No, definitely not." We were relieved. I wanted to make sure she was happy living with us.

Her room was down the hall from our kitchen, and she would often ask me what I was making for dinner. I would tell her it was something good, but not as good as when she made it. Mom was a fantastic cook and terrific baker. Believe me, everything she made was the best.

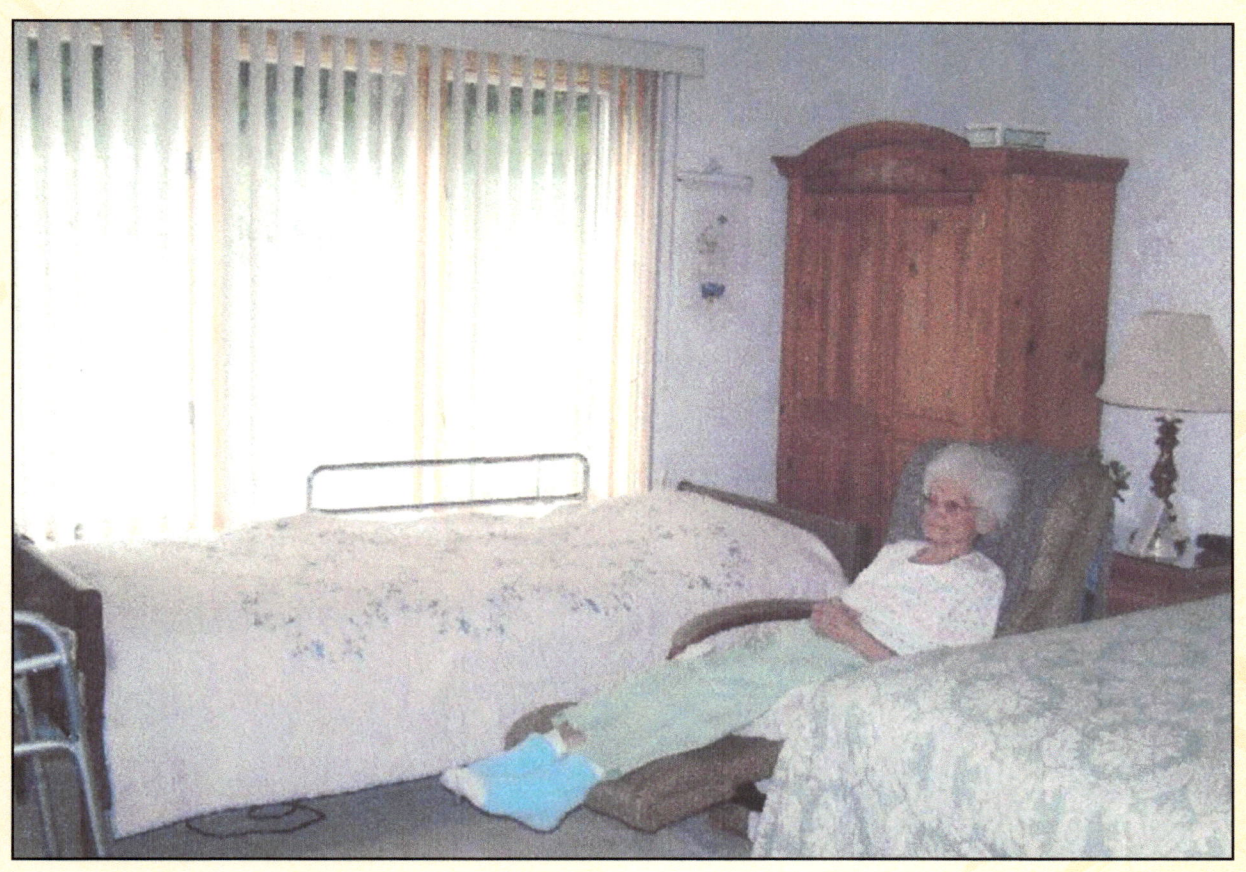

In the beginning, Mom and I would play card games, watch television together, and talk about the old times. There were days when she wouldn't know who I was and days when she would remember everything and everyone. Thank goodness, she would always know her son, my husband, and they always had great memories to talk about. I loved listening to them talk and joke about everything.

When we would watch television together, she would often ask me who the actors were and their names. There were times when we would just talk, and I would put my hand on her arm. She would pick up my hand and kiss it. I was deeply touched and knew she was grateful to be living with us and not in a nursing home.

When Mom first came to live with us, we had hospice in the beginning and then again at the end. Words cannot describe what a great organization they are and how truly wonderful are the nurses and the girls that work for them.

From time to time, I had assistance from caregivers from a local agency. They were all wonderful girls and so dedicated.

I worked two days a week for a great orthodontist. On these days, my husband took care of Mom by himself. When I came home from work, she would say, "Where were you all day? I missed you."

I will always be grateful to my husband for also wanting to keep his mom in our home. Without each other, we could not have taken care of her.

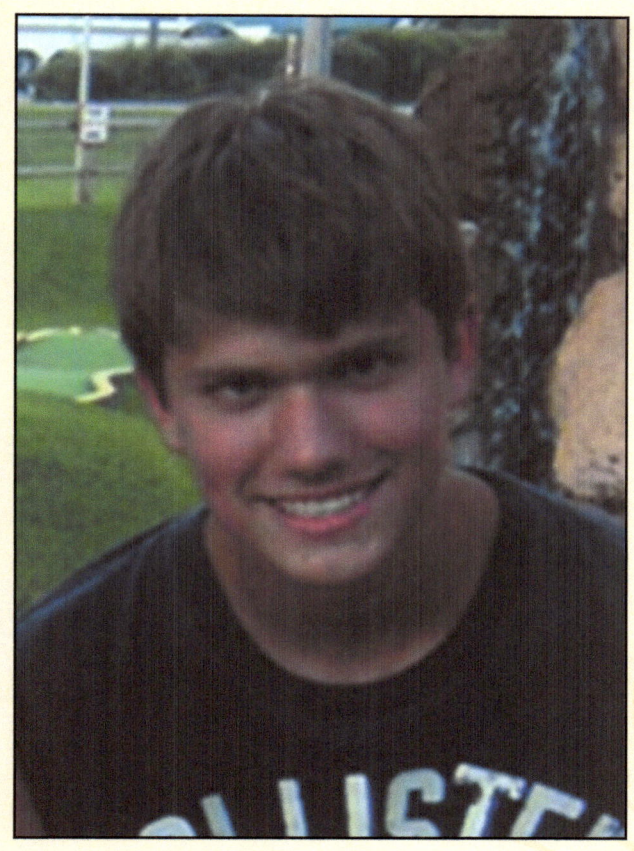

Tyler

We are so grateful to our children, who helped us whenever we needed them.

Our grandson Tyler, who was in high school then, came over almost every night to help put Mom in bed. She used to babysit him, and now he was helping her.

Mom always loved when her great-grandchildren came over. They entertained her by pretending to fix her wheelchair, playing with blocks on the bed, or just watching TV with her.

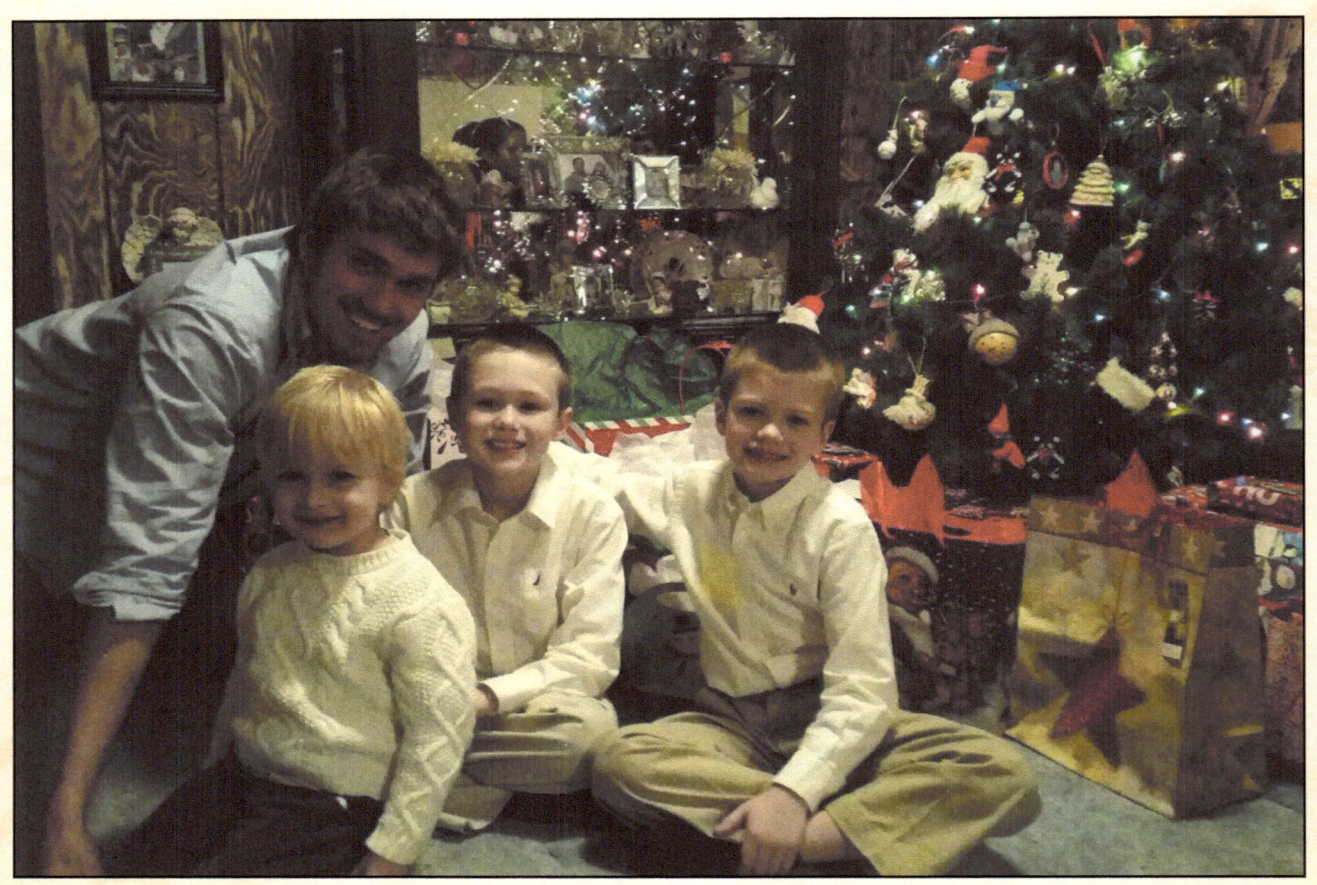

Tyler, Montgomery, Austin, and Landon

Mom used a walker at first, which helped her a great deal. After a while, Mom rubbed her heels (as she slept) into blisters and then sores. After months and months of us going to the wound clinic and having them cleaned and dressed every night, her heels got better.

The doctor and girls at the wound clinic were wonderful and so helpful. This was when I heard about special medical bootees for Mom's feet (these I should have had the first day she came to live with us). After her heels healed, we started therapy to get her to walk again, but it was in vain. It was just too hard for Mom to walk again.

Another item we needed was a hospital bed with an inflatable mattress. This helped her keep from getting bedsores.

We needed a seat or chair in the shower. This made it easier for her and for us.

A wheelchair was also a tremendous help. After her heels healed, she was unable to walk or even stand. She depended completely on us to pick her up from the bed to the wheelchair and to the shower.

Creams and lotions were so important and necessary to keep her skin soft, which helped prevent sores.

Gauze and bandages were a necessity. There were times when she would rub off the skin on the tops of her feet by rubbing on the wheelchair foot holders. When we picked her up to transfer her from the bed to the chair, her feet tended to drag, which caused the skin on her toes to open. They needed to be cleaned and covered every day.

We also needed incontinence supplies, bed-protection pads, and a gel seat for the chair our loved one sat on daily.

My husband always took care of all the medication and vitamins she needed daily. He took time each weekend to create a list and organized them in pill containers for the week.

Having a television in her room was really helpful. It kept her company when we were doing other things.

There are so many other things you can't possibly get out of books. You need to feel them inside as you go along and work them out.

Someone once said to me that we dragged out her life by taking good care of her. A very wise nurse told me we gave meaning to her life by not putting her in a nursing home, because she would have lived as long as God wanted her to live and not one second less.

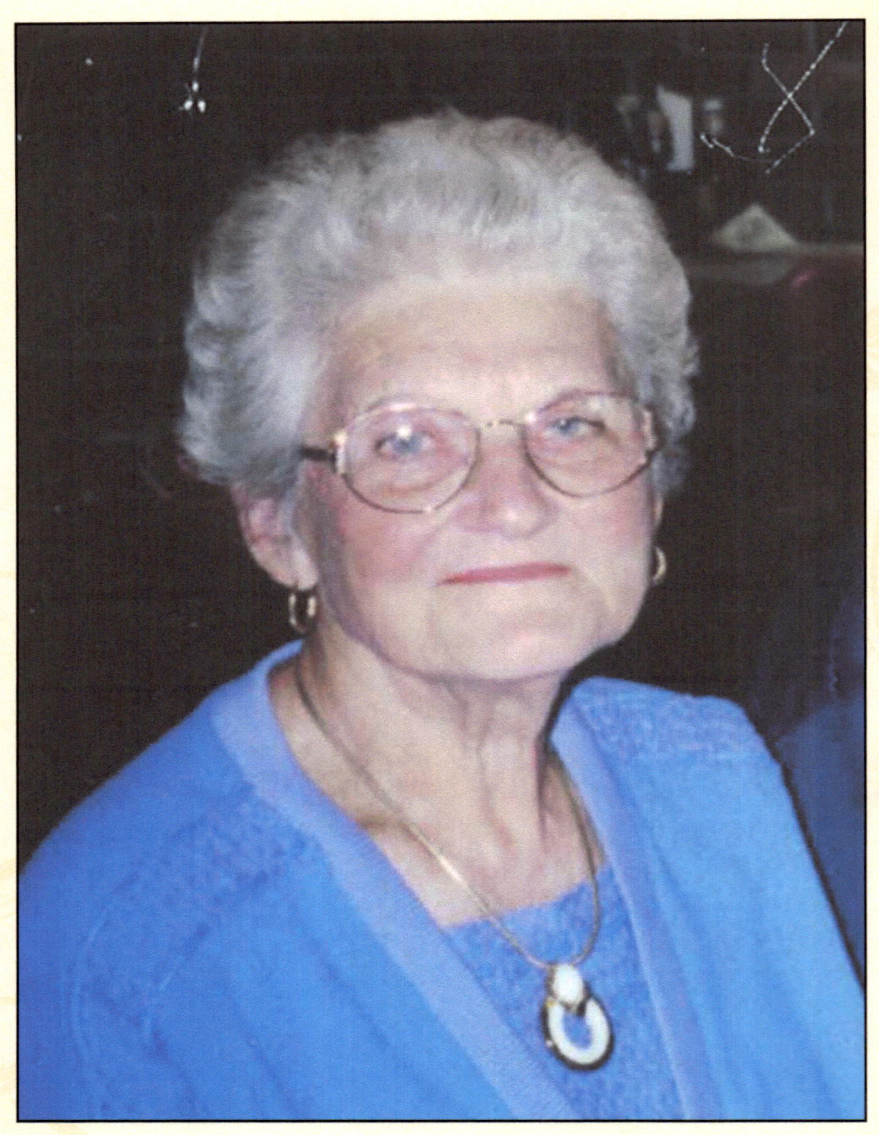

Mom died on July 29, 2013. She was ninety-three years old. We still can't believe she is gone. We miss her so much.

The day after she died, she came to me in a dream. She looked beautiful. She kept shaking her head and saying, "I can't believe you kept me for four and a half years." I knew she was with God and it was her way of saying, "I'm okay, and thank you for keeping your promise."

Take care of your parents. You owe your life to them. I know not everyone can take care of a loved one, but if you can, it's an amazing journey.

To review, here are the items we believe you may need in caring for an elderly loved one:

1. Medications and vitamins

2. A walker

3. Medical bootees for their feet

4. Gel pad for their chair

5. Hospital bed with an inflatable mattress

6. Incontinence supplies

7. Mattress-protection pads

8. Creams and lotions

9. Wheelchair

10. Seat/chair in the shower

11. Gauze and bandages

And last but not the least, you need patience and love.

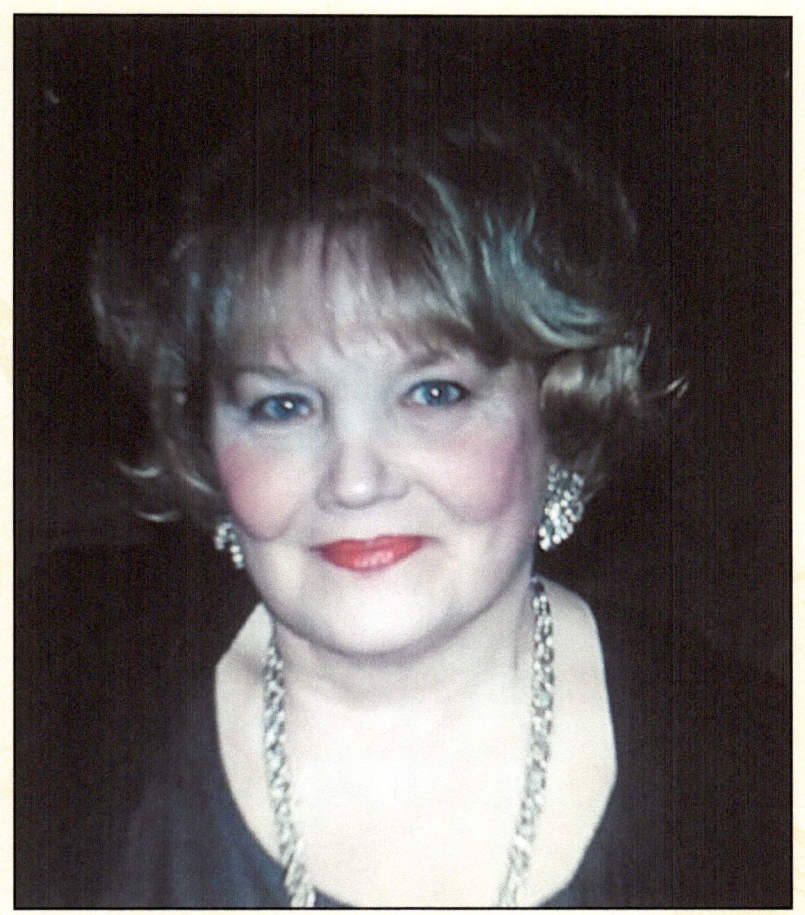

D. J. Aust

You never know what is going to happen in life or when you are called upon to keep a promise.

We were so blessed by God to have her in our lives. Taking care of Mom has changed our lives. I hope this book changes yours.